God Made Food For You and Me

Matthew Strohhacker, MBA, MPH, CPH
Karena Strohhacker, APRN, MSN, AGACNP-BC

For permissions or inquiries, contact:
Karatt Multimedia, LLC.
Website: karattmultimedia.com
Email: karattmultimedia@gmail.com

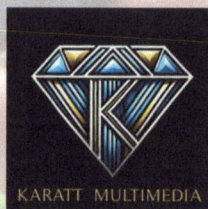

KARATT MULTIMEDIA

ISBN: 978-1-971047-00-3
Printed in the USA.

To Elle, Carter & Joel,
May God bless you with a lifetime of
health, purpose, passion
and His unending favor.
You are deeply loved – always & forever!

To every child, parent & mentor,
May you embrace the gift of
health and inspire others
to grow into their best selves,
all through the loving hands of God.

To _____

- M.S. & K.S.

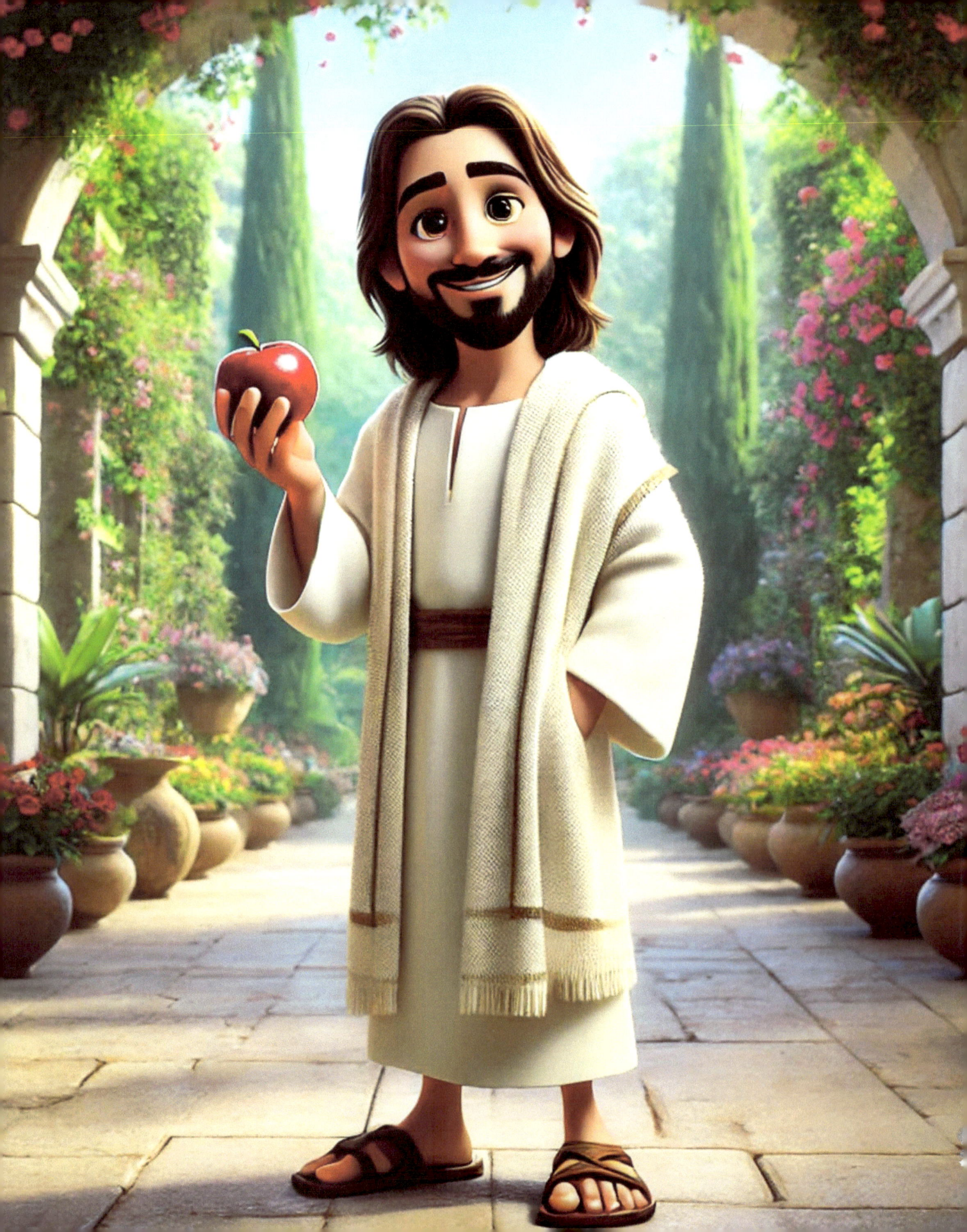

God made apples,
red and sweet.

A crunchy snack,
a perfect treat!

They help your heart
grow strong and true—

So you can run, jump
and play too!

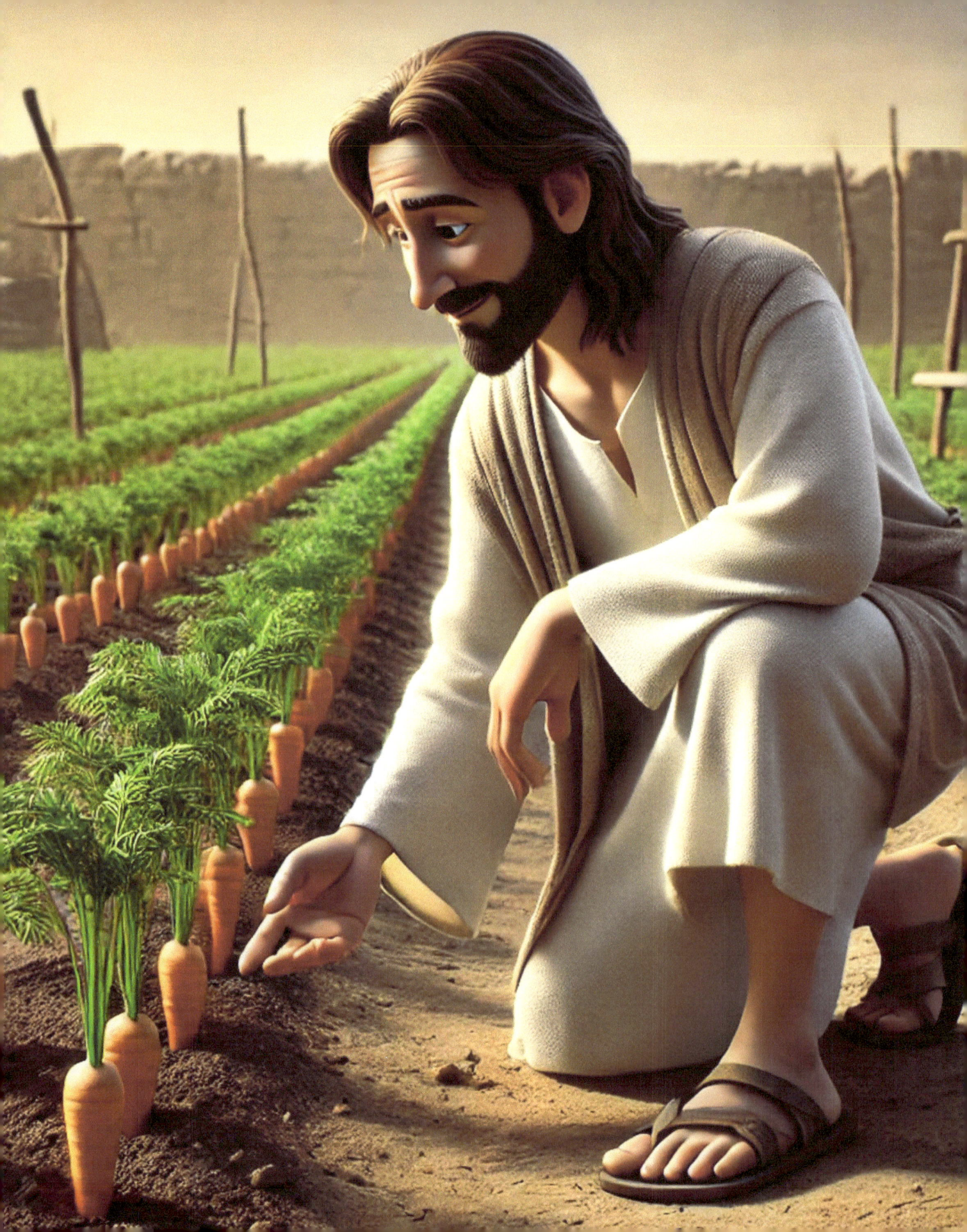

God made carrots,
orange and bright.

Helping your eyes
see in the light.

They show the
world's wonders,
far and near—

Every color, crystal clear!

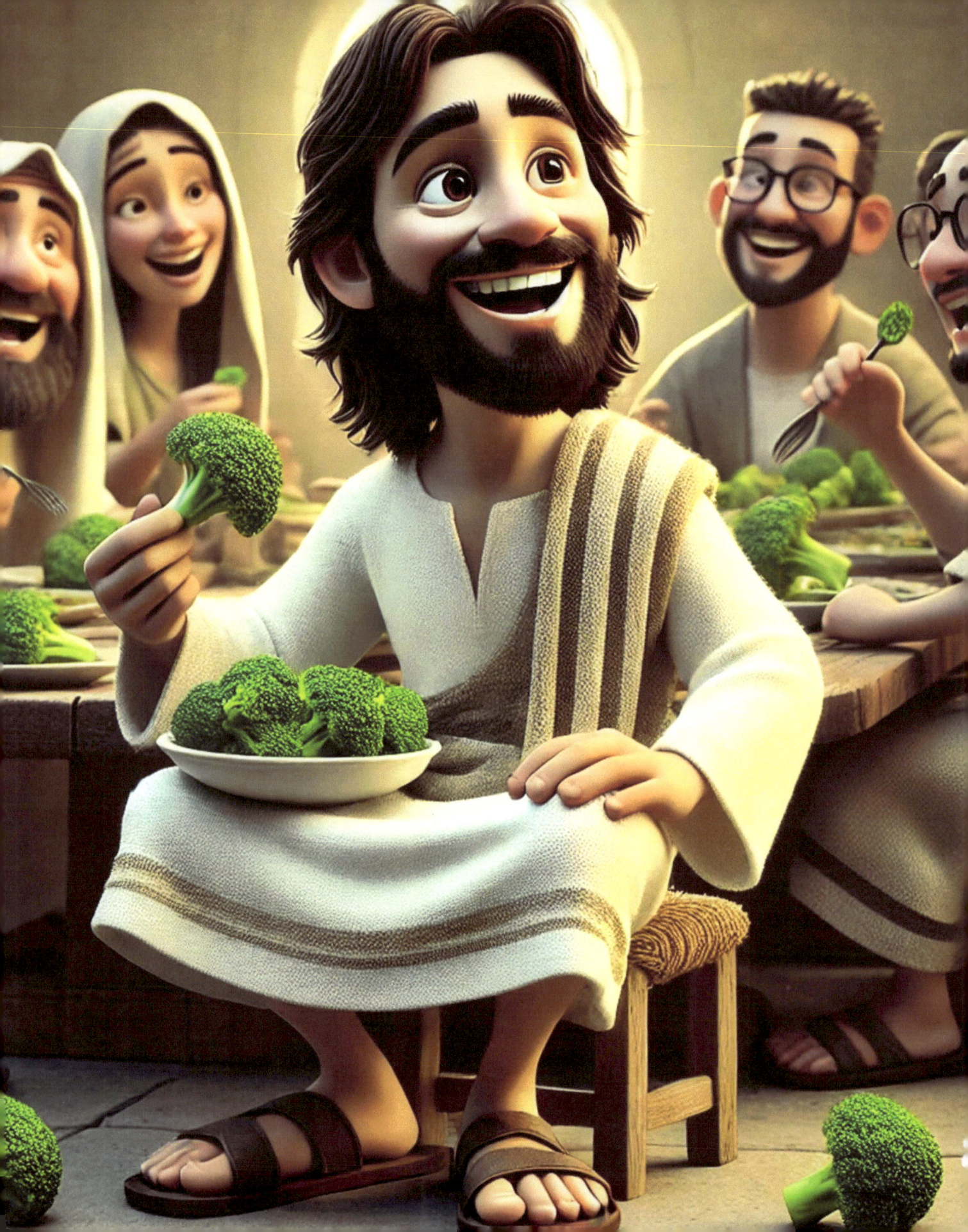

God made broccoli,
green and small.

Tiny trees for one and all!

It gives you strength
to jump and grow—

And keeps your body
in tip-top flow!

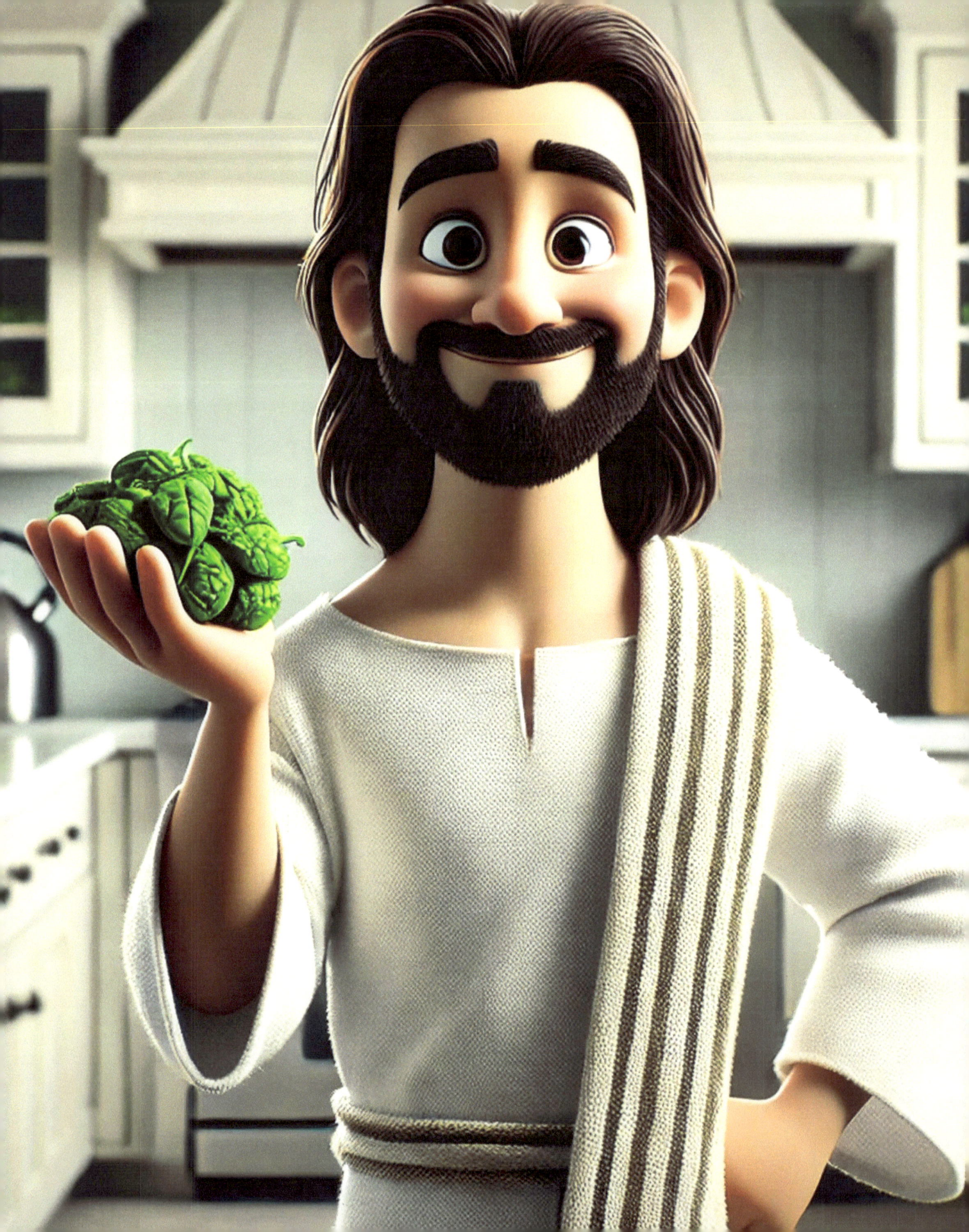

God made spinach,
leafy and green.

For muscles as strong
as you've ever seen.

Climb and lift,
carry and play—

Spinach helps you every day!

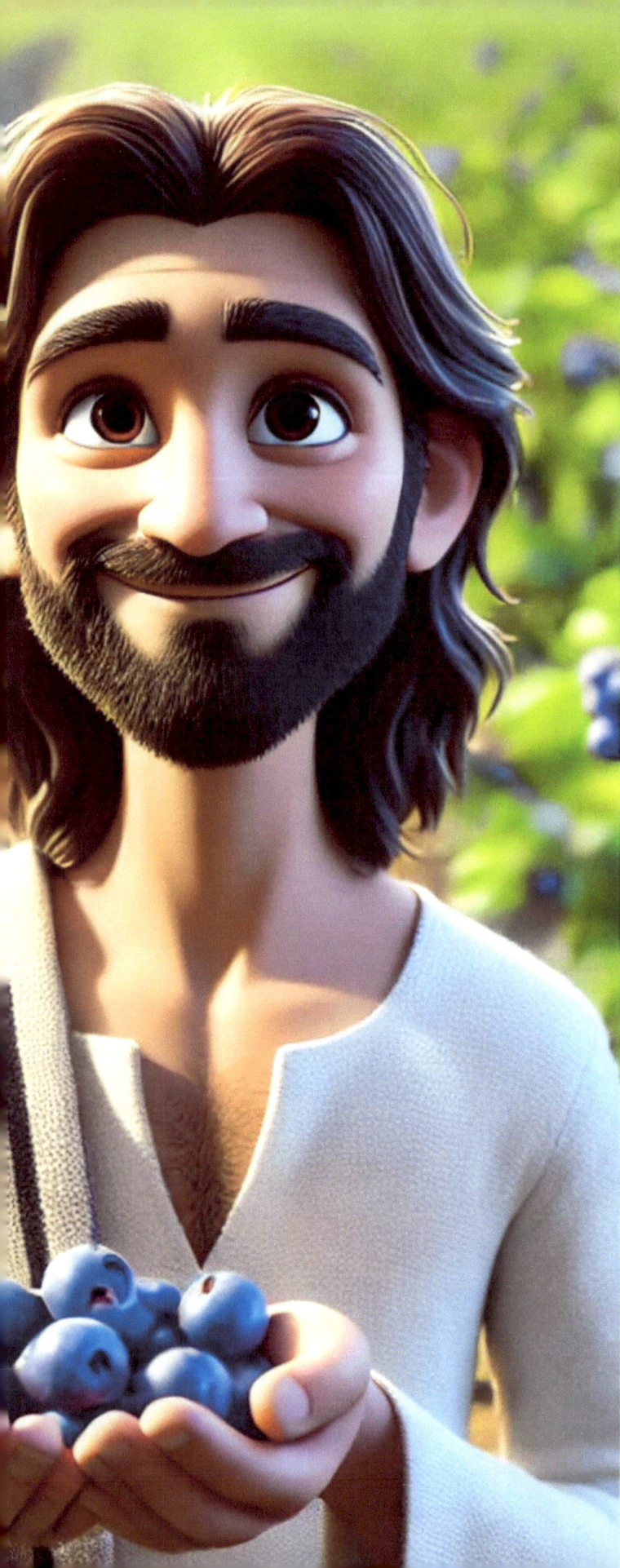

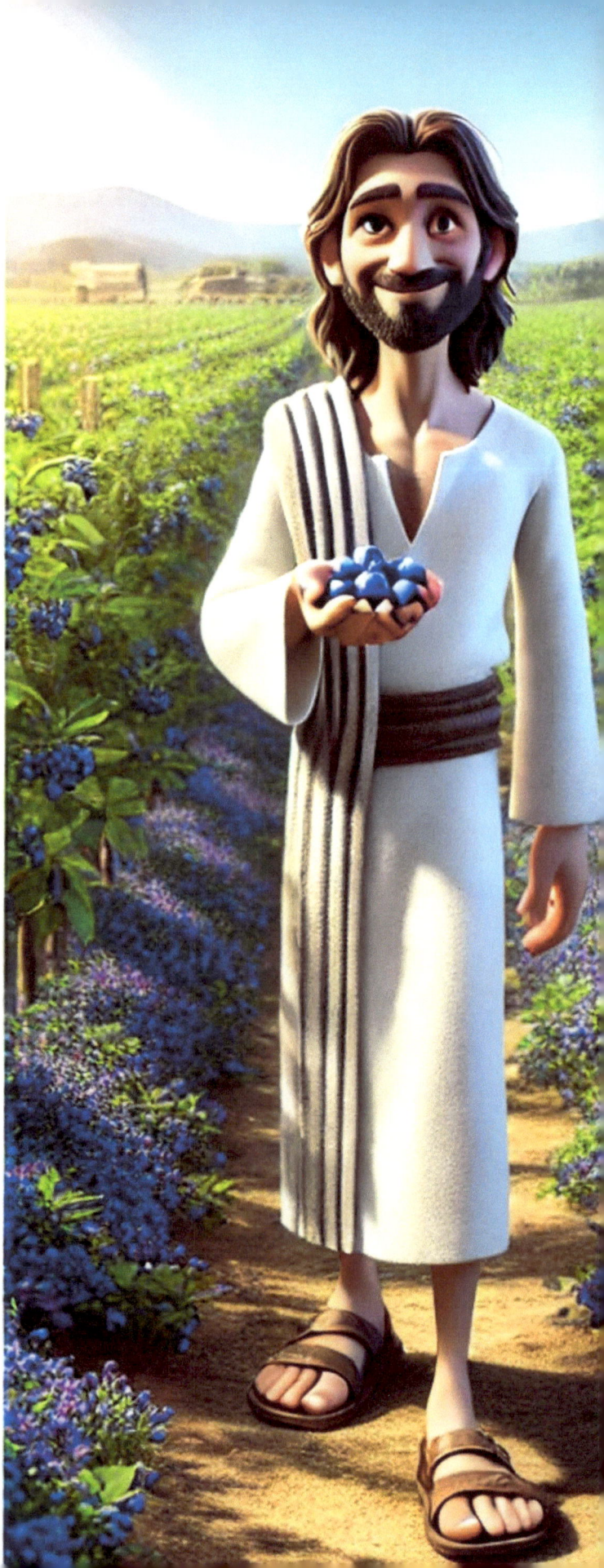

God made blueberries,
little and round.

Little brain boosters
growing on the ground.

They help you think,
they help you learn.

New ideas at every turn!

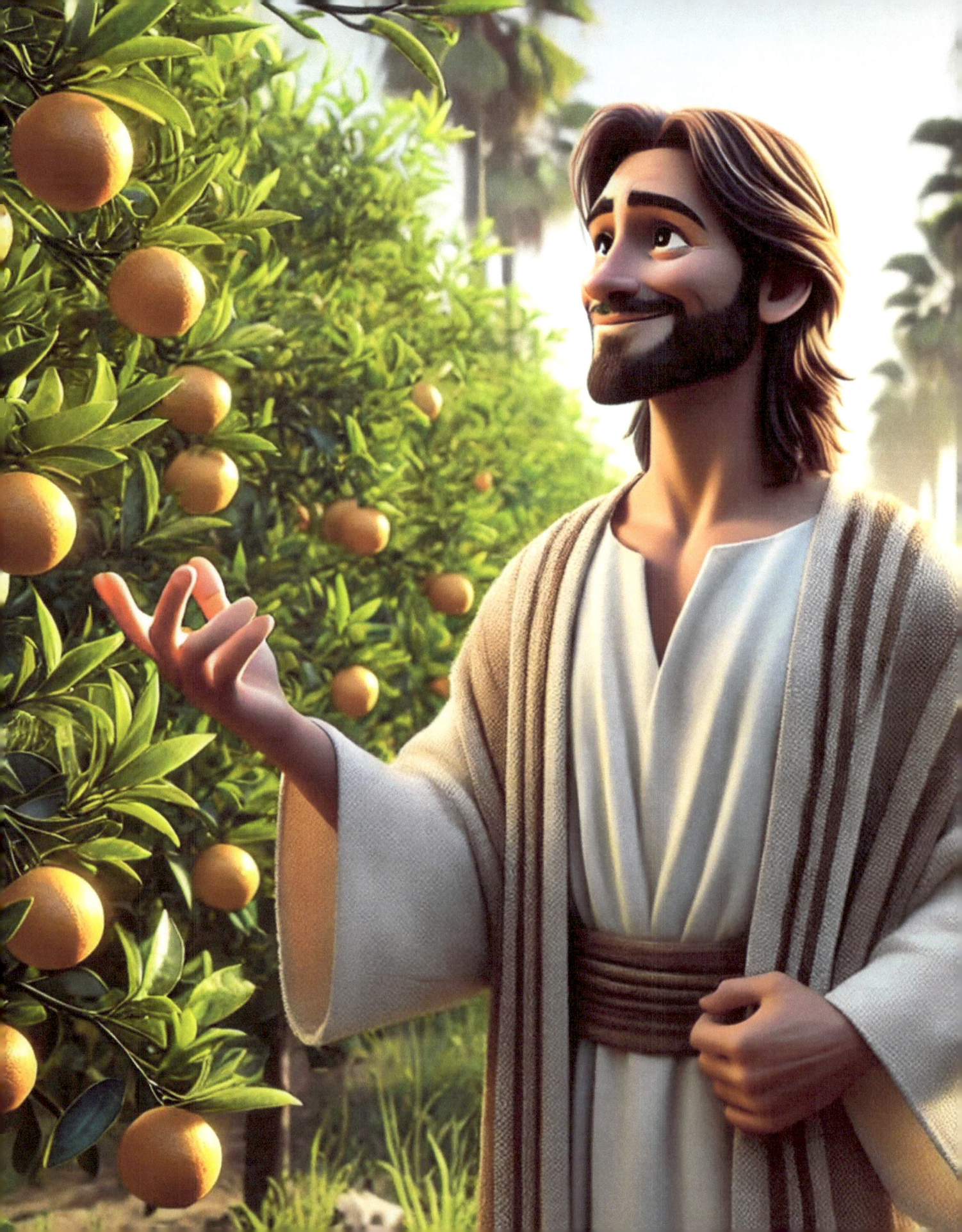

God made oranges,
juicy and bright.

Filled with sunshine,
pure delight!

With vitamin C,
they help you stay-

Healthy and happy,
come what may.

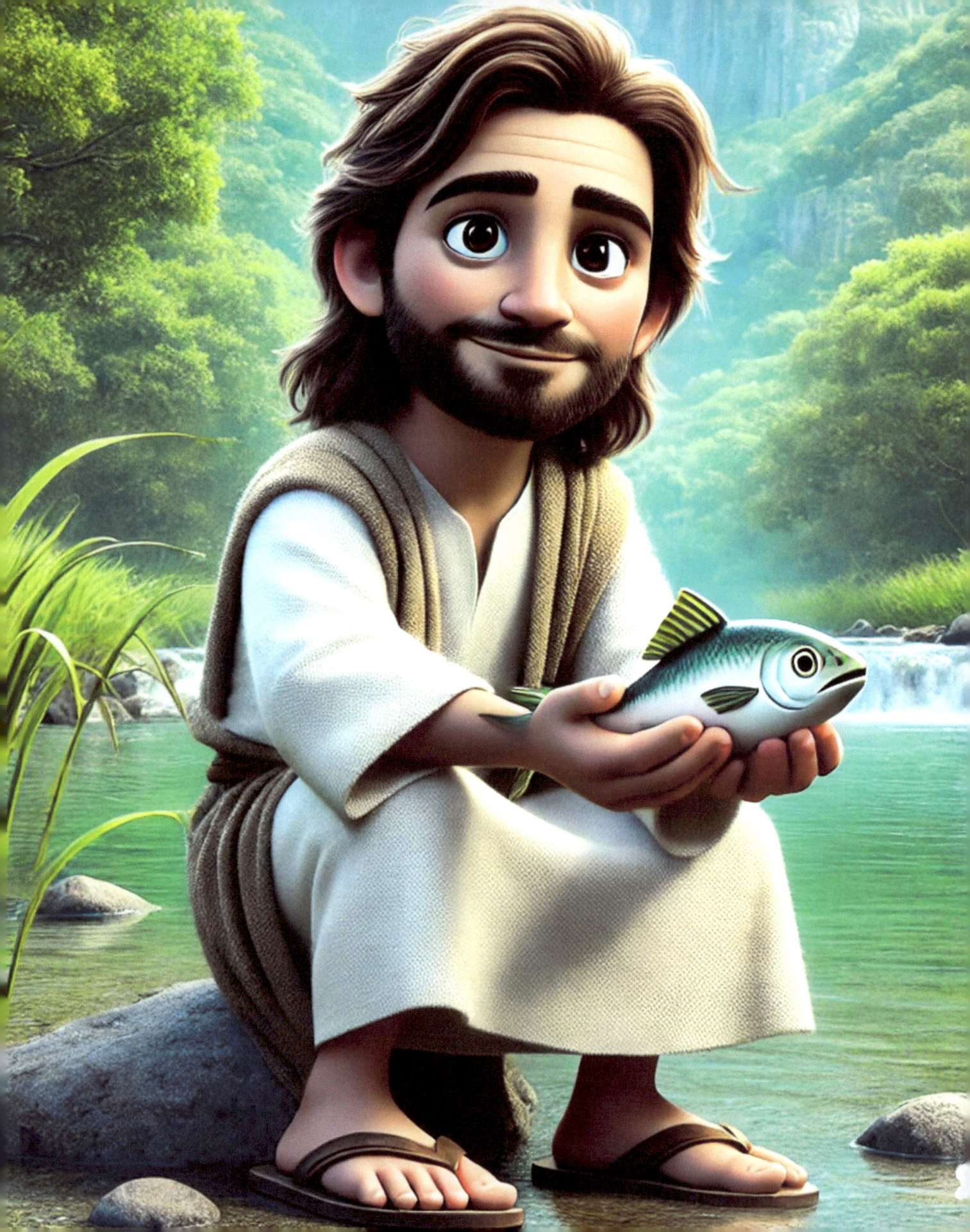

God made fish
that swim in the sea.

With omega-3s
for you and me.

They make our brains sharp,
quick, and clear-

To solve, imagine
and persevere!

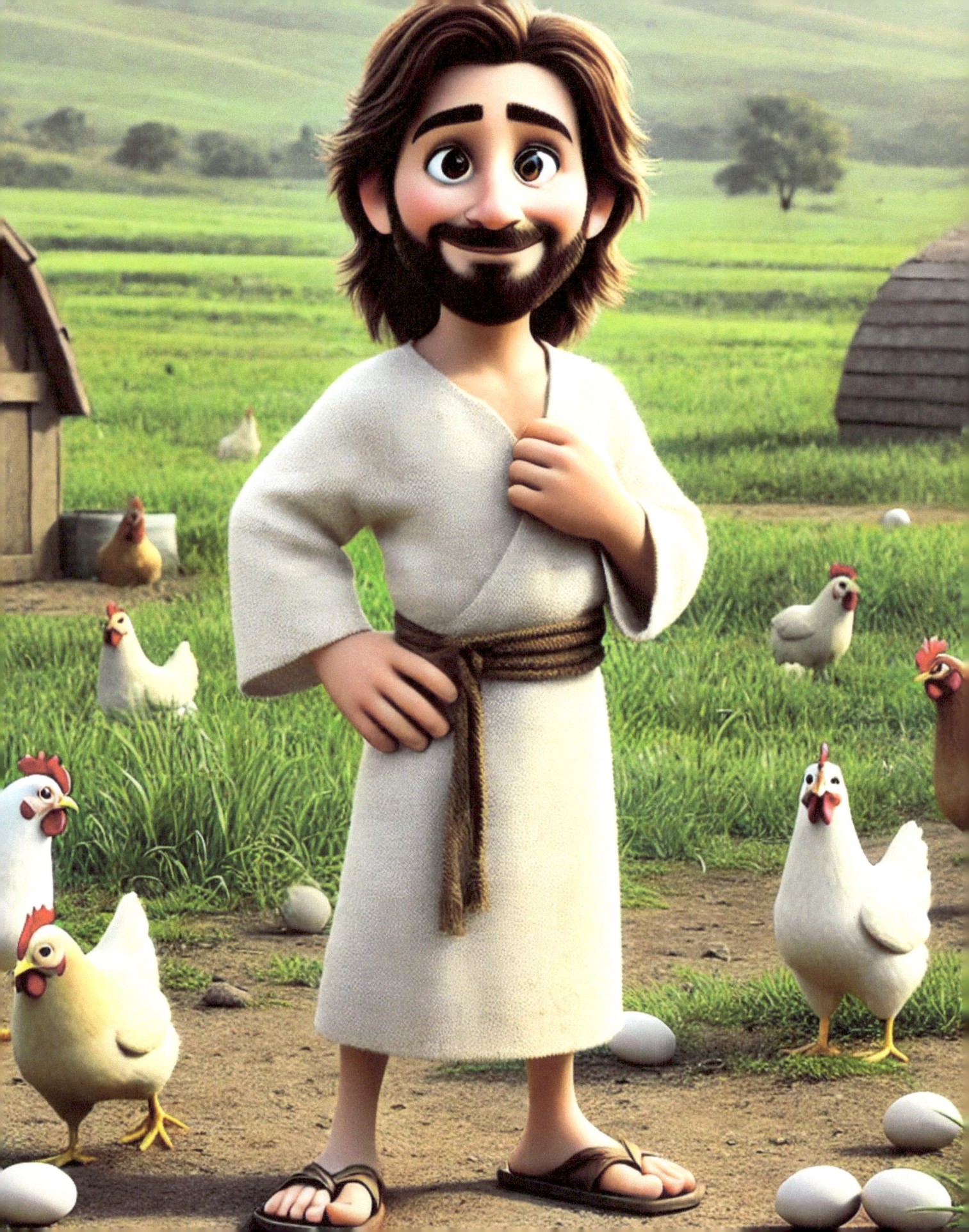

God made eggs,
a protein prize.

To help you grow
and energize.

They build you up,
from head to toe—

Eggs help your body
bloom and grow!

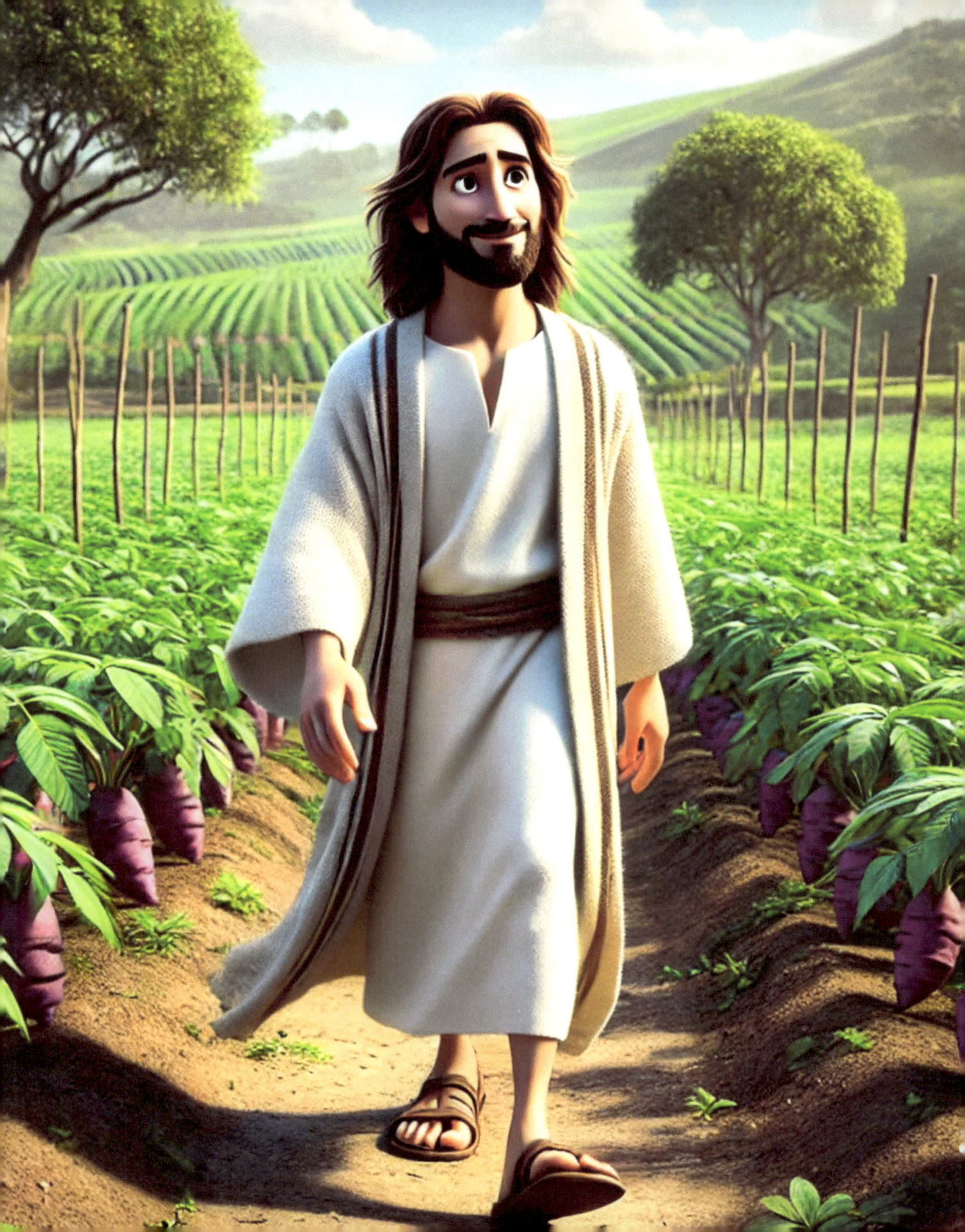

God made sweet potatoes,
orange and sweet.

There's energy in
every bite you eat.

They power your day,
keep you on your way-

From morning sun
to evening play!

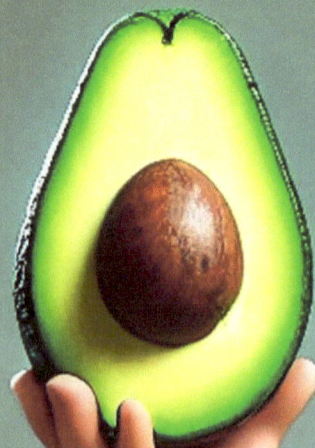

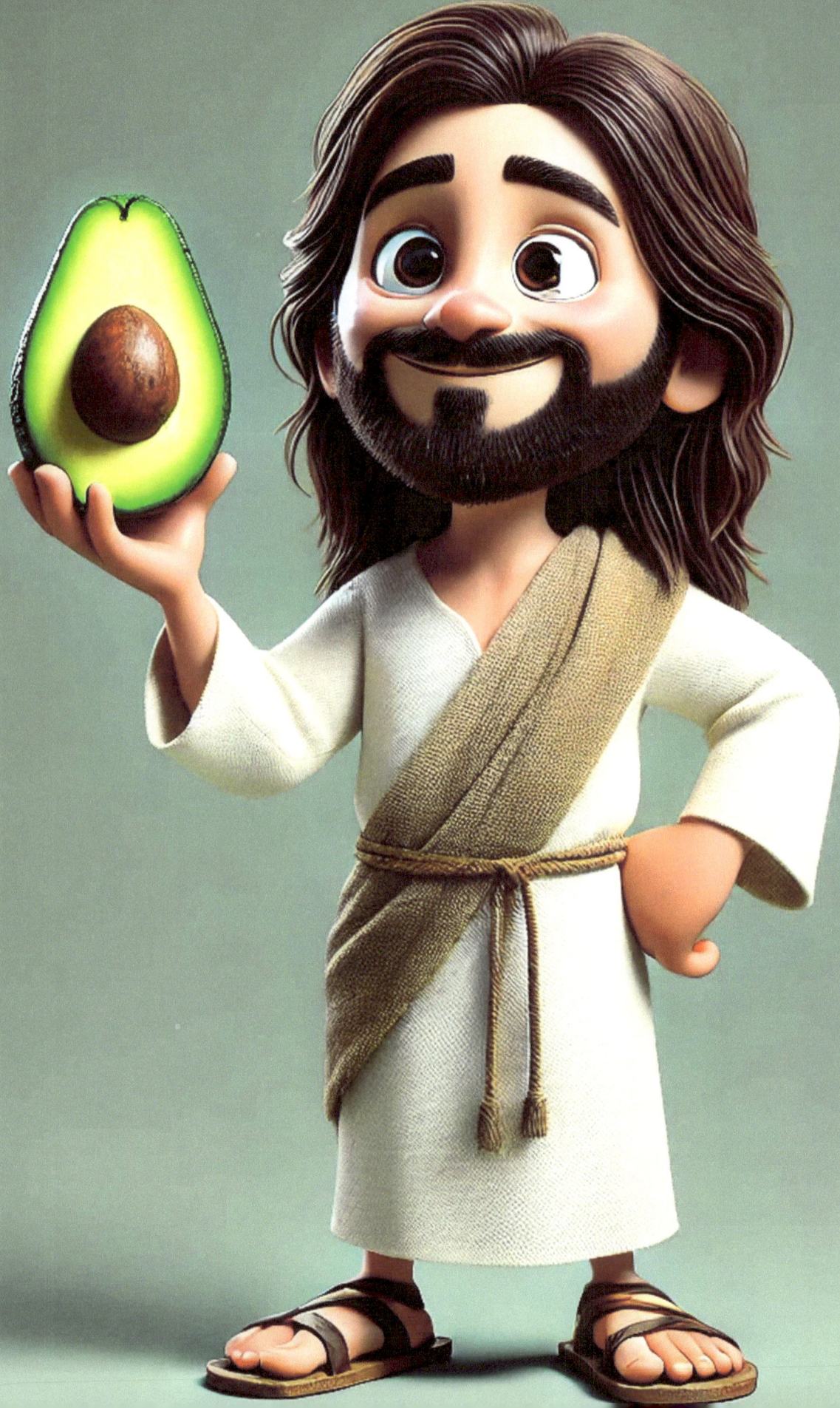

God made avocados,
green and creamy.

A fruit so rich,
it feels so dreamy!

It helps your heart
and makes your skin glow.

A gift from God
to help you grow!

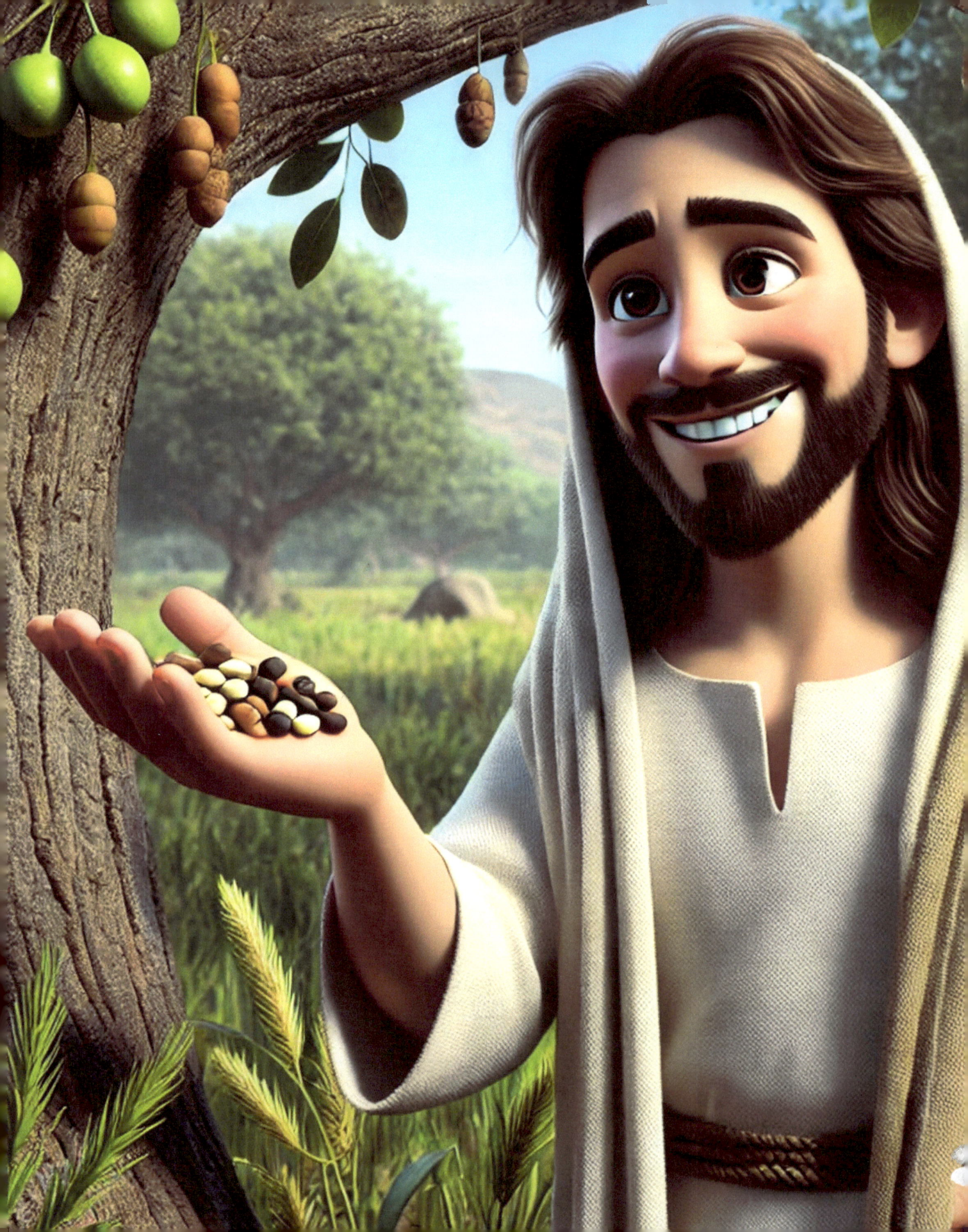

God made nuts
and seeds so small.

But they're packed with
strength to share with all.

Crunchy bites
to help you stay-

Full of energy,
for work and play!

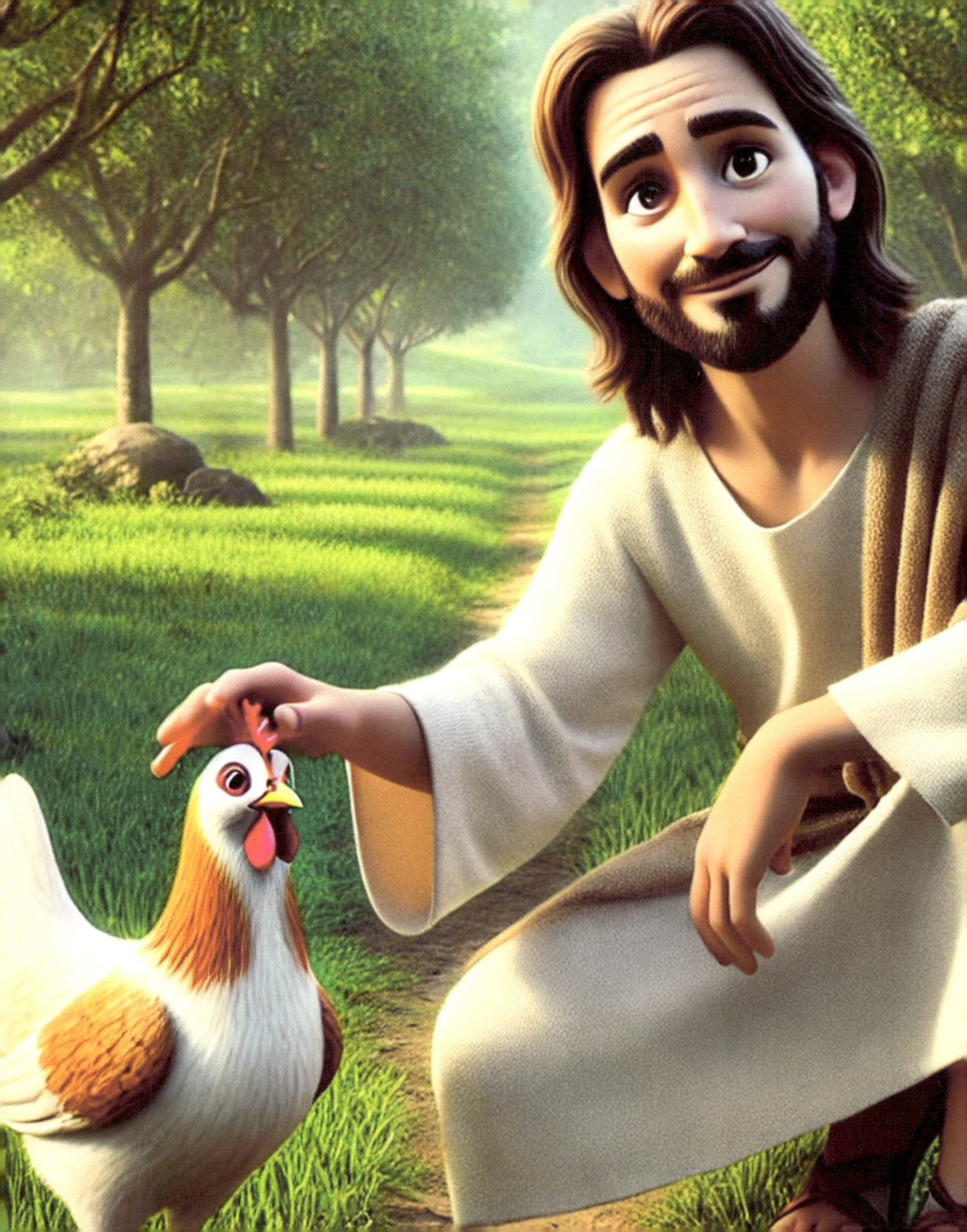

God made chicken,
tasty and lean.

A muscle-builder
that's pure and clean.

It helps you run, jump,
skip and glide-

And keeps your
body strong inside.

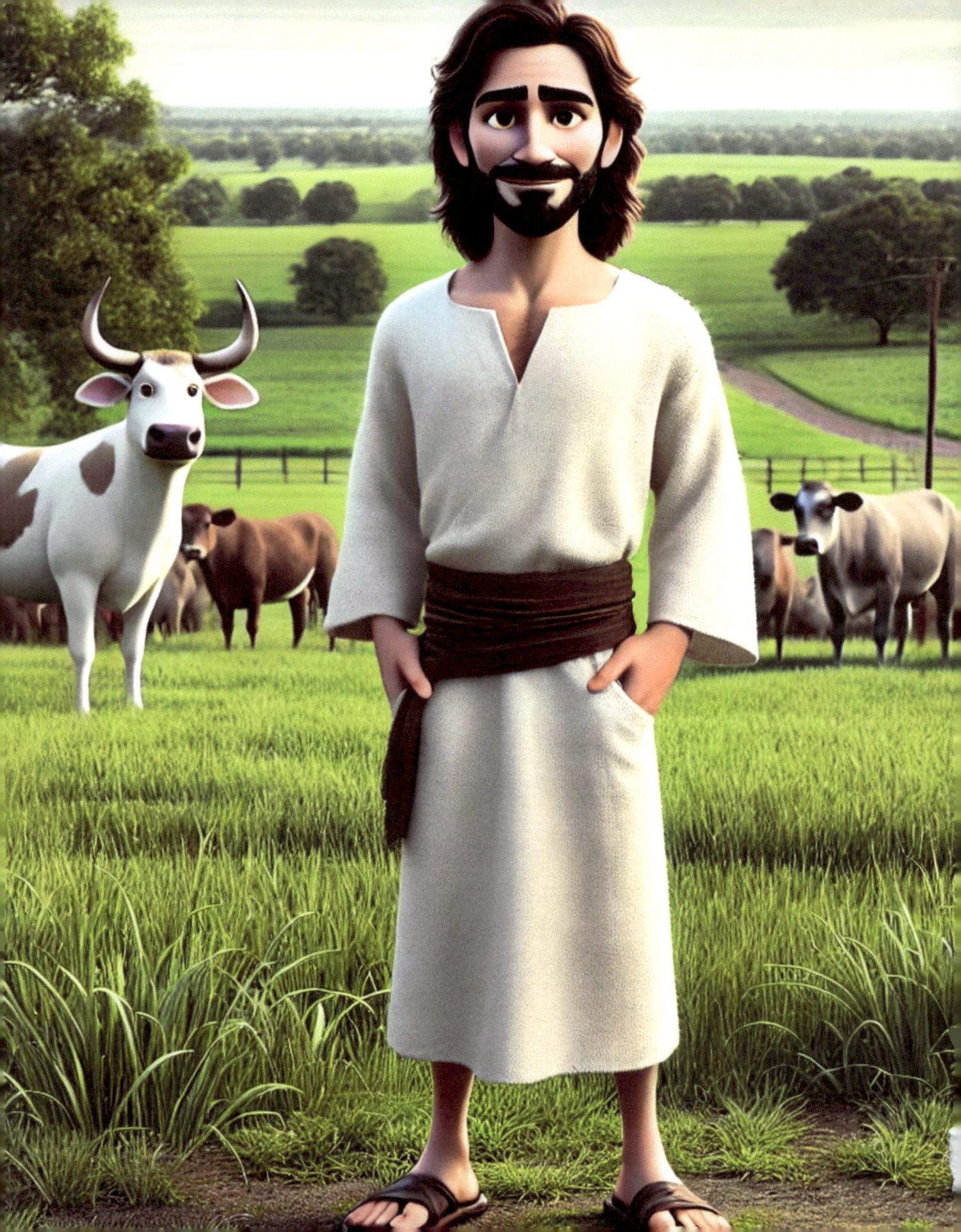

God made cows
and beef so sweet.

Rich in iron,
a hearty treat!

It keeps you strong,
it keeps you bold—

With energy that
you can hold!

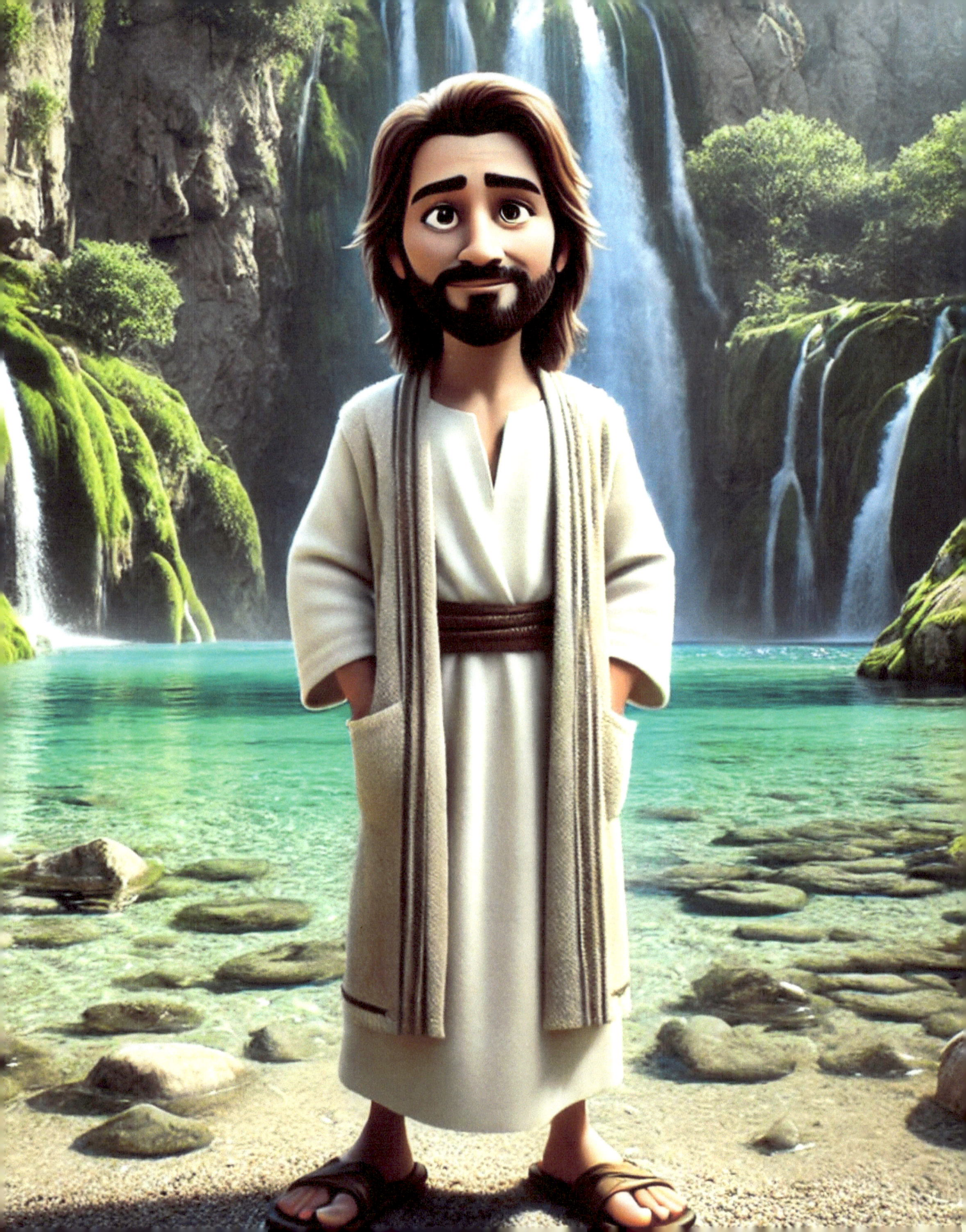

God made water,
clear and bright.

To keep you healthy,
day and night.

Every cell needs
water to glow—

Drink up, and let
your energy grow!

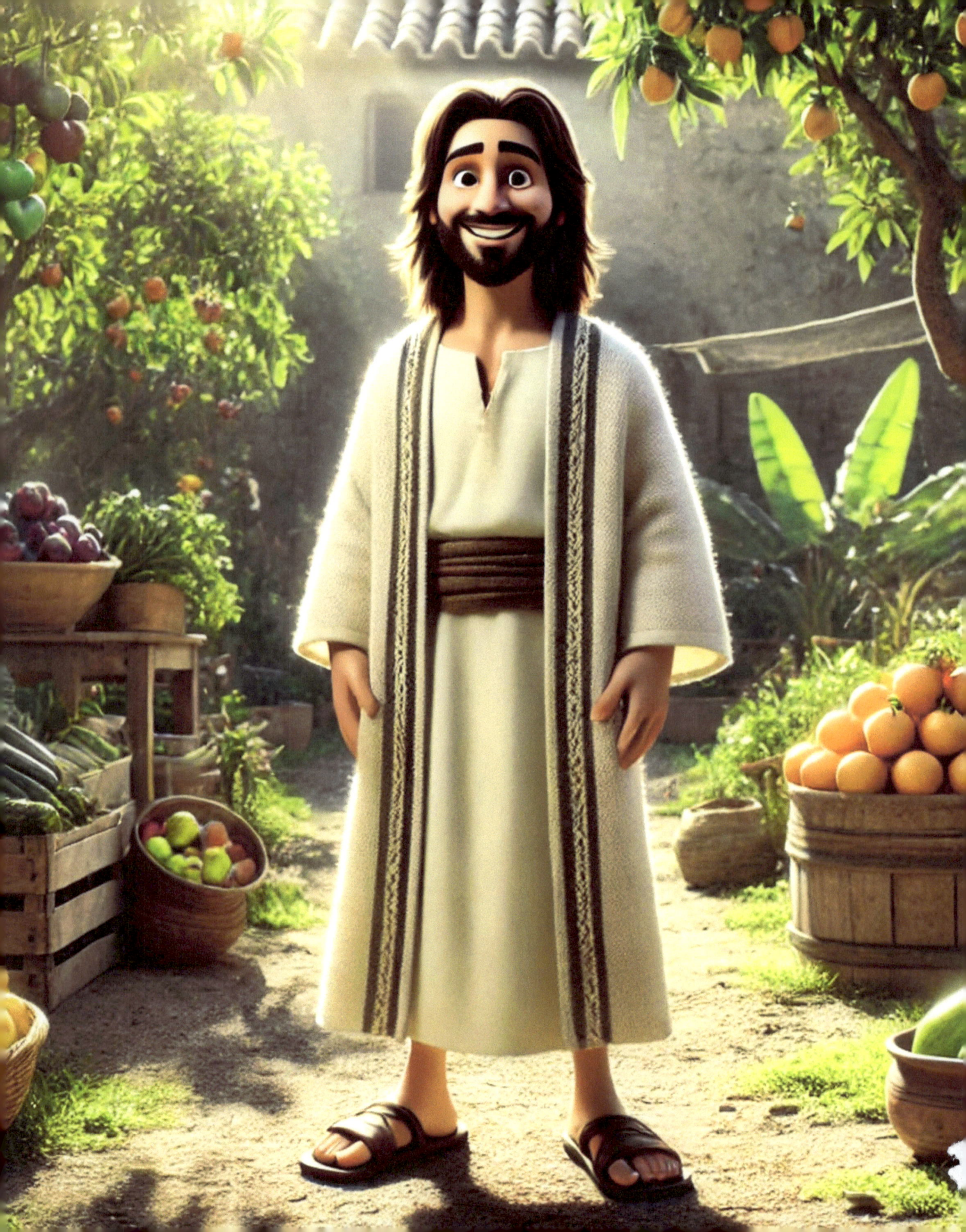

God made the sun,
warm and high.

Helping plants grow
toward the sky.

It gives us vitamin D
for our bones—

And fills the day
with golden tones.

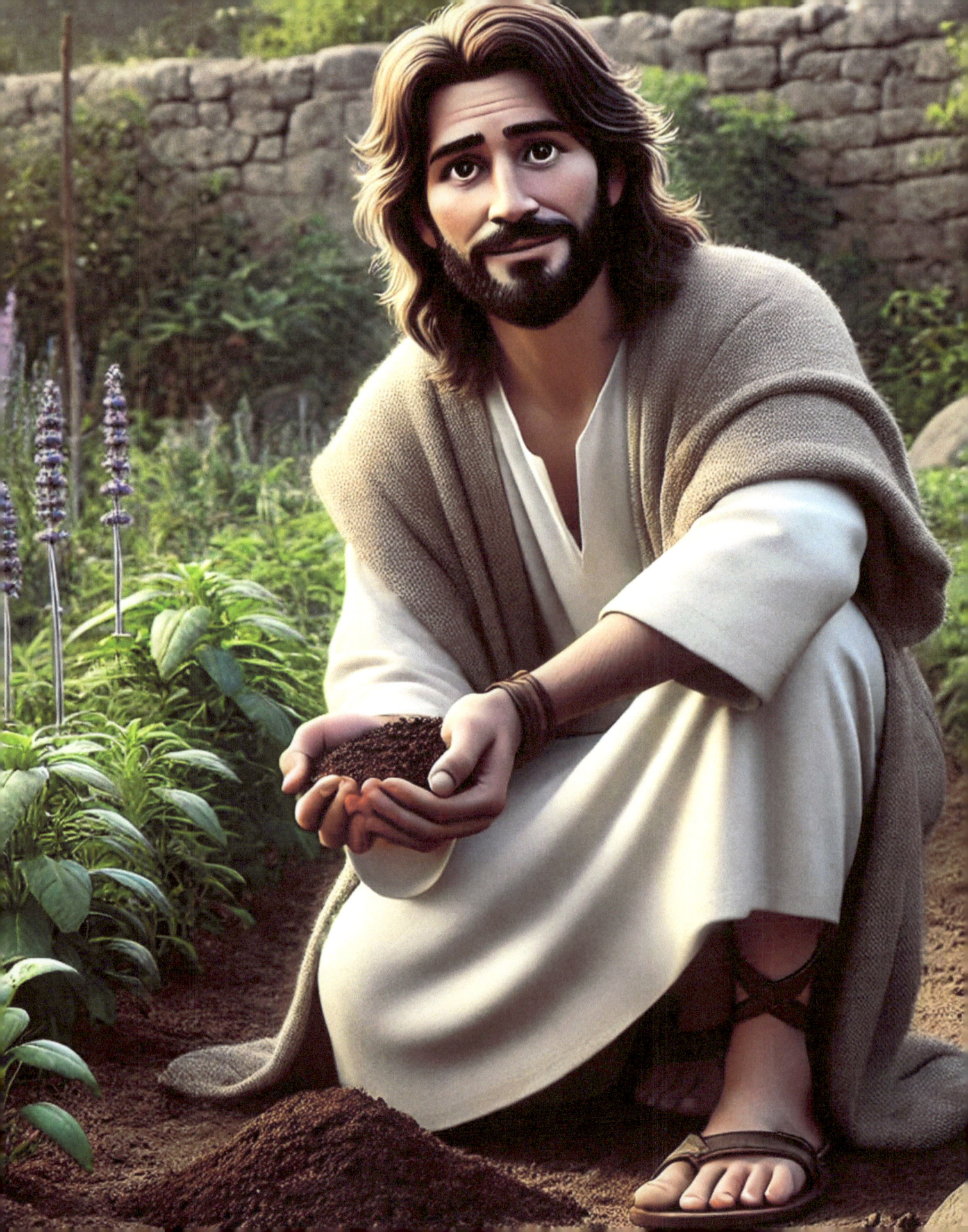

God made soil,
dark and deep.

Where fruits and veggies
love to sleep.

Full of nutrients,
rich and true.

The soil helps them
grow for you!

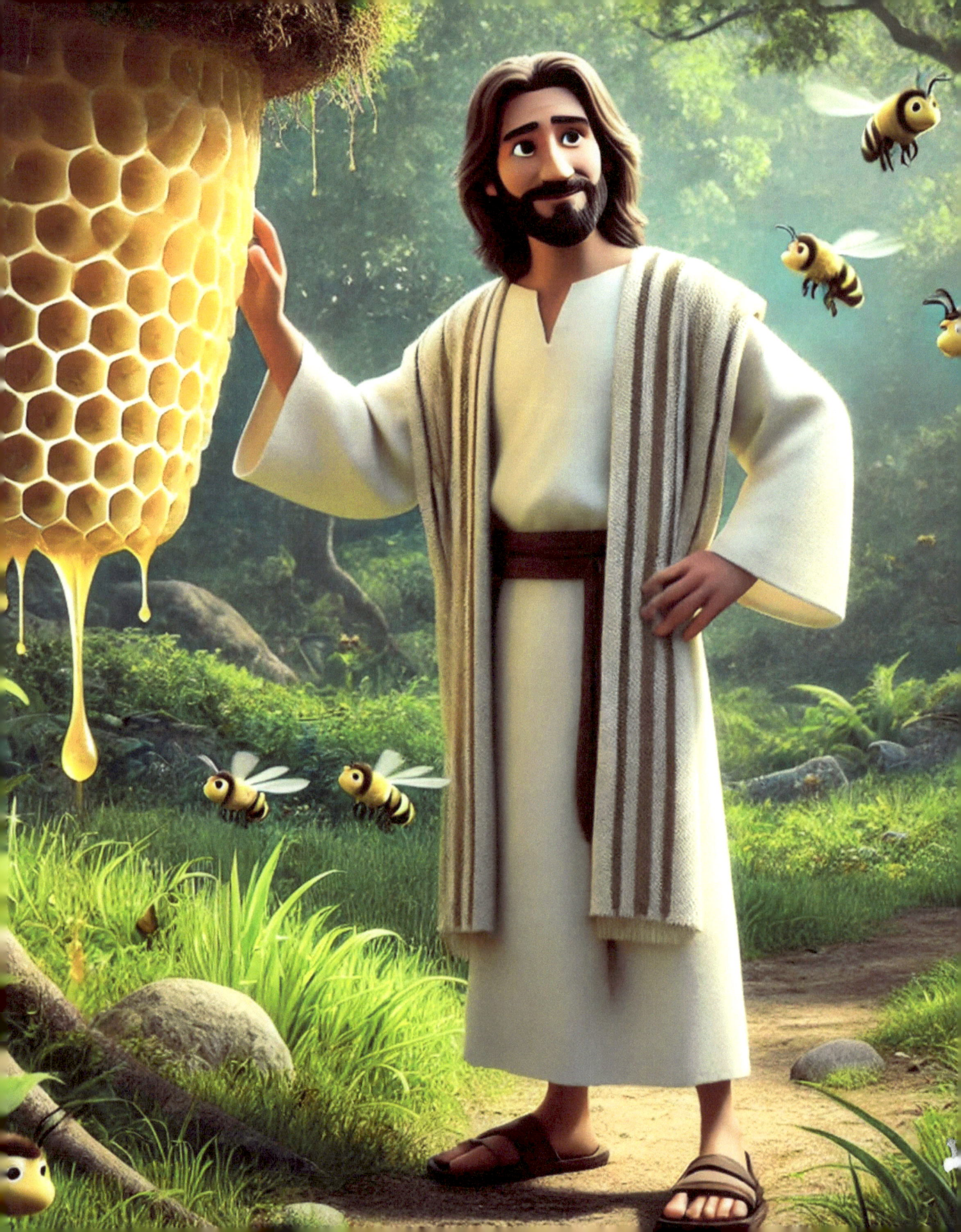

God made honey,
golden and sweet.

A buzzing bee's
delightful treat!

It gives us energy,
smooth and light.

And makes each day
taste just right!

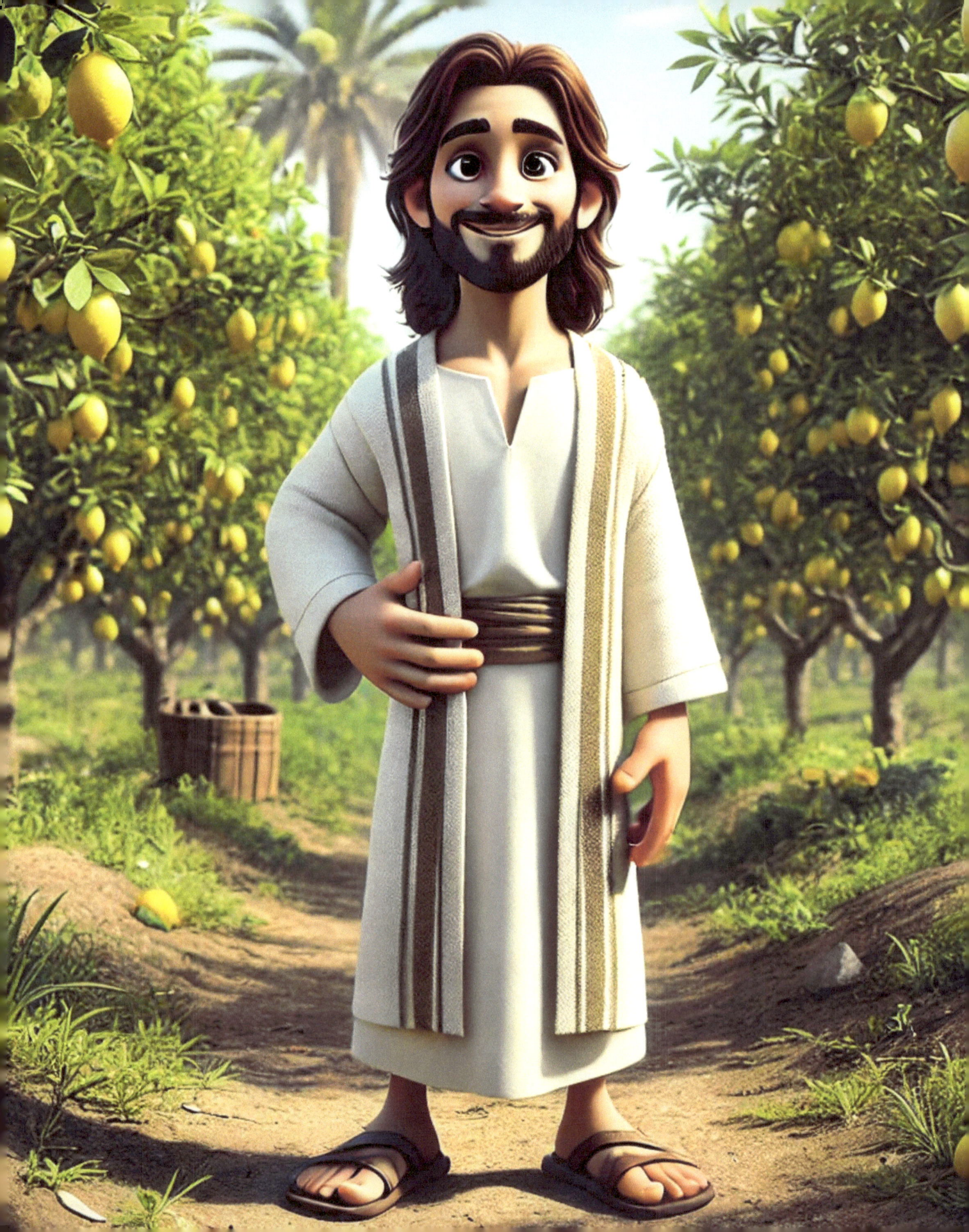

God made lemons,
bright and sour.

A tart fruit with
cleansing power.

A little squeeze
in water or tea.

Keeps you feeling your best,
you'll see!

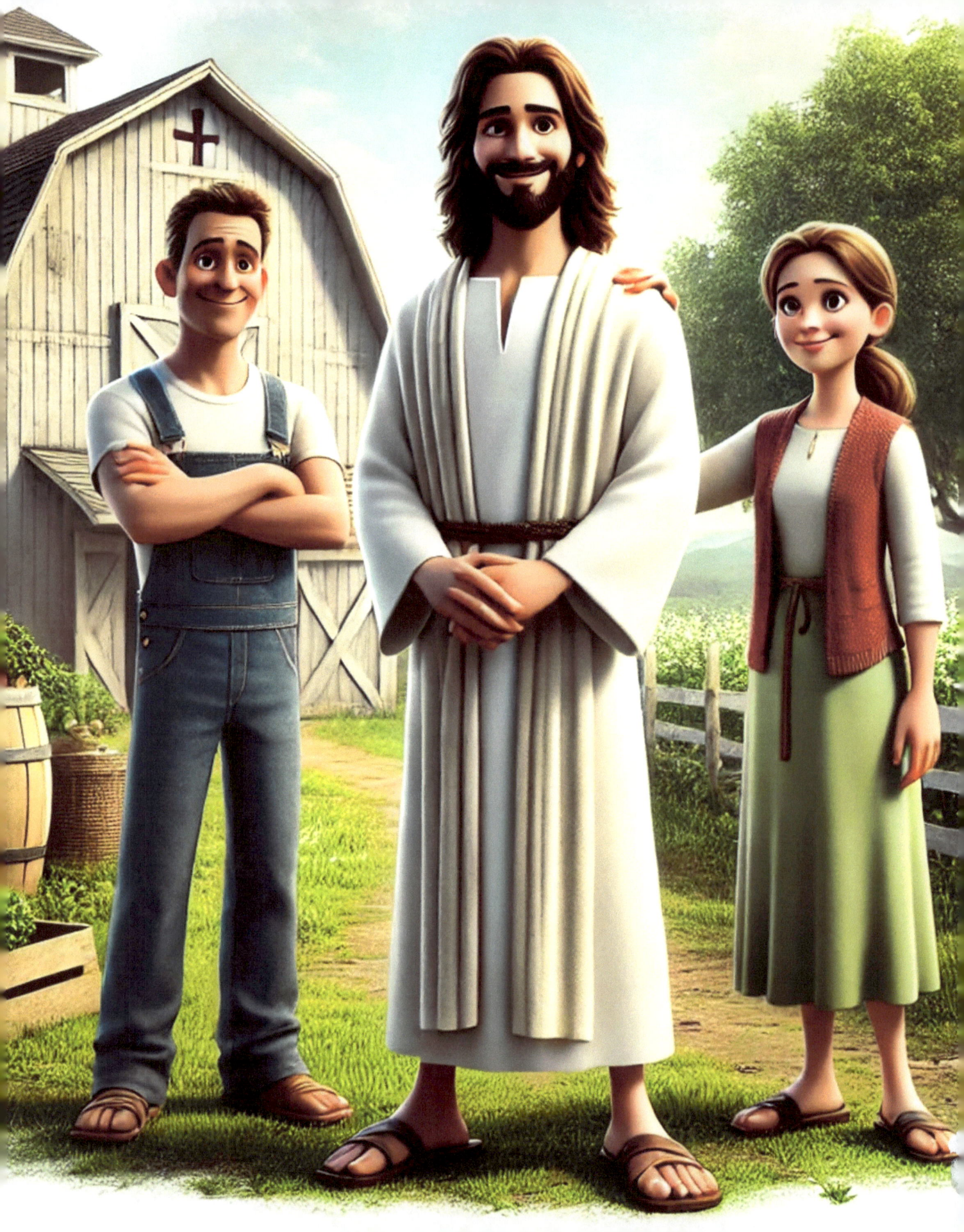

God made farmers,
working the land.

Planting seeds with
a caring hand.

They bring us food,
they tend and sow.

So we can thrive and
grow and grow!

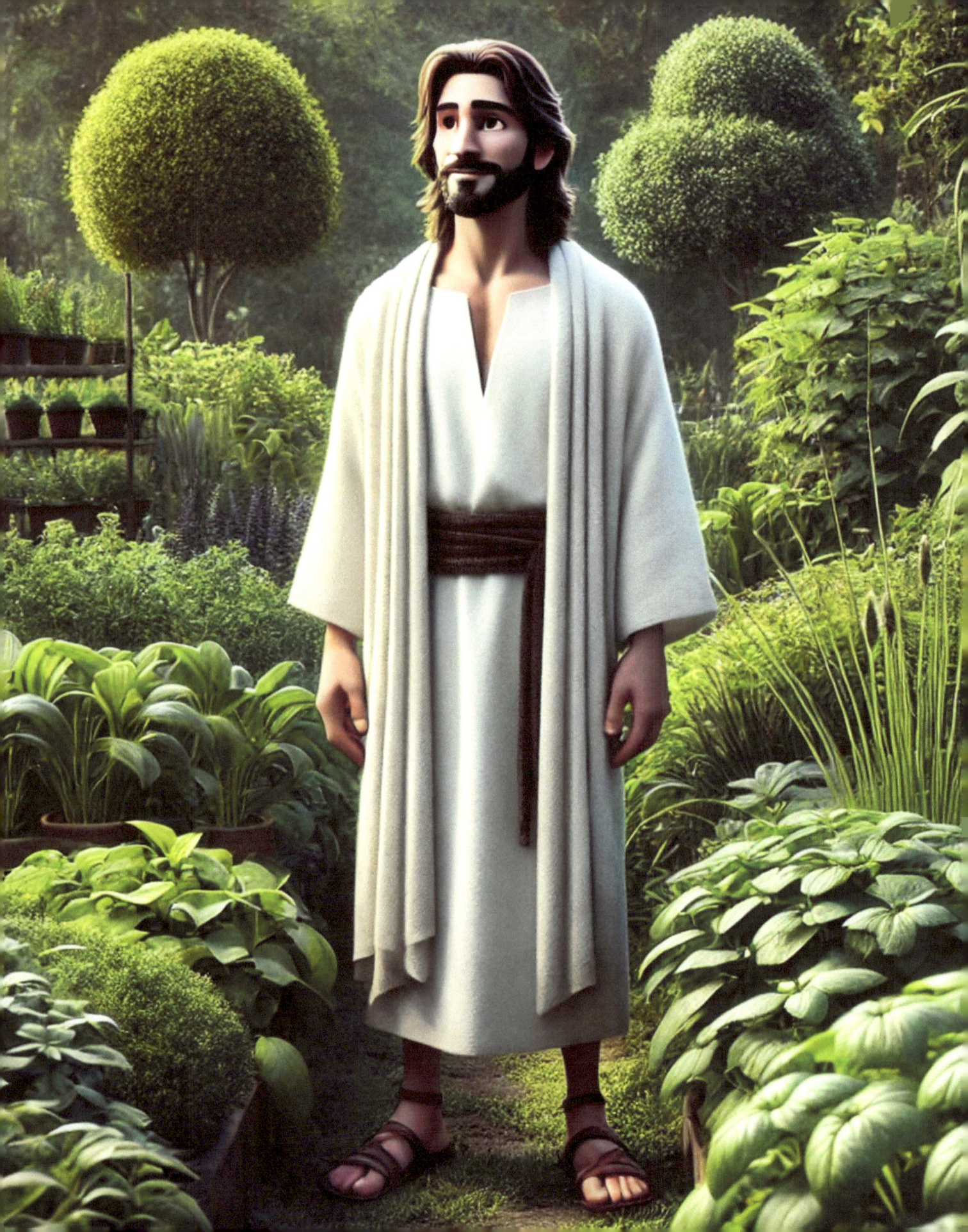

God made herbs,
like mint and thyme.

To make our meals
taste oh-so-fine.

They calm our tummies,
add flavor too—

A sprinkle of herbs
is good for you!

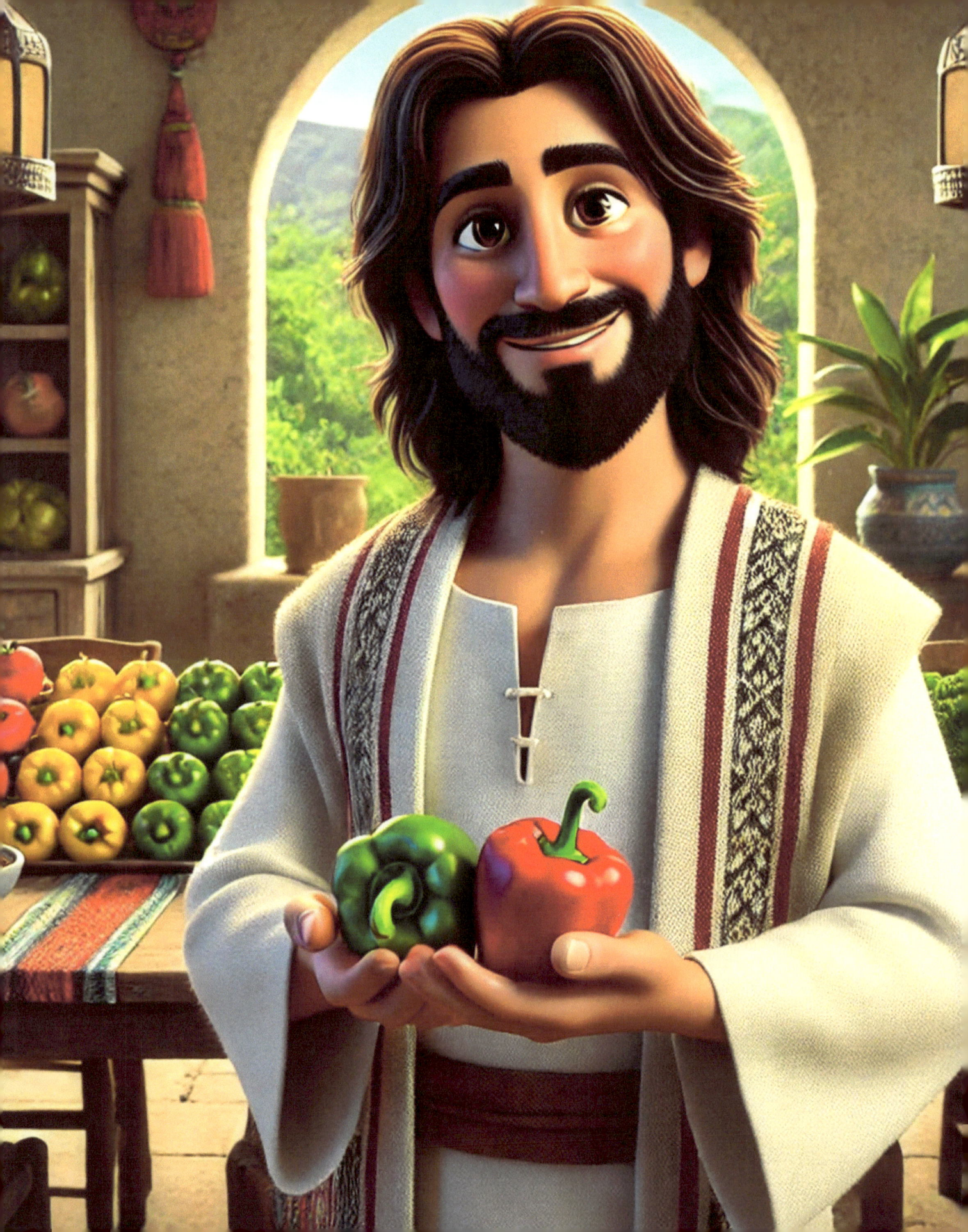

God made peppers,
red, yellow, green.

Bright as rainbows,
a colorful scene.

They help your skin
and hair stay strong.

And add a crunch to
meals all day long.

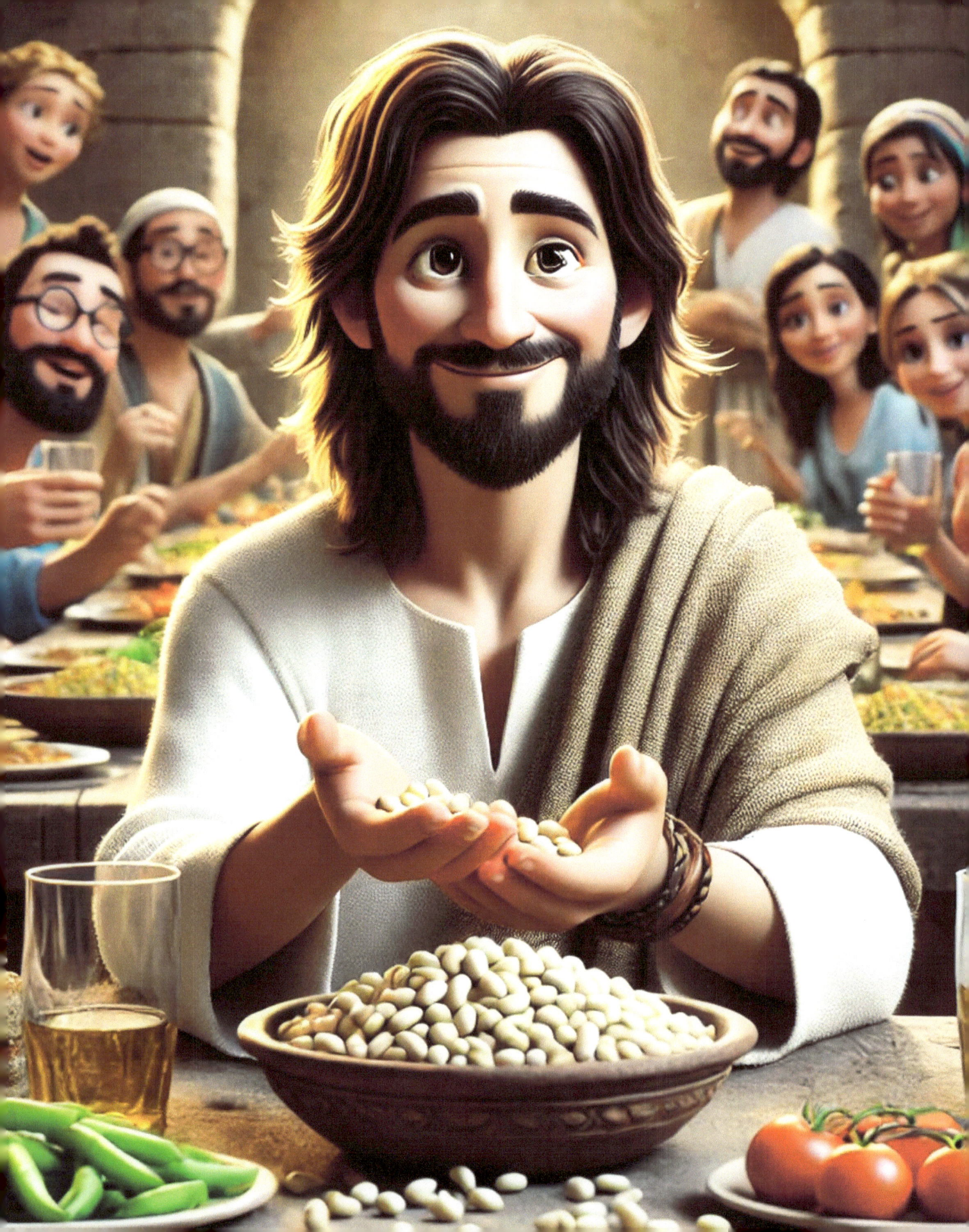

God made beans,
a powerful snack.

Packed with goodness,
they've got your back.

They fill you up
and keep you going.

With every bite,
your strength is showing!

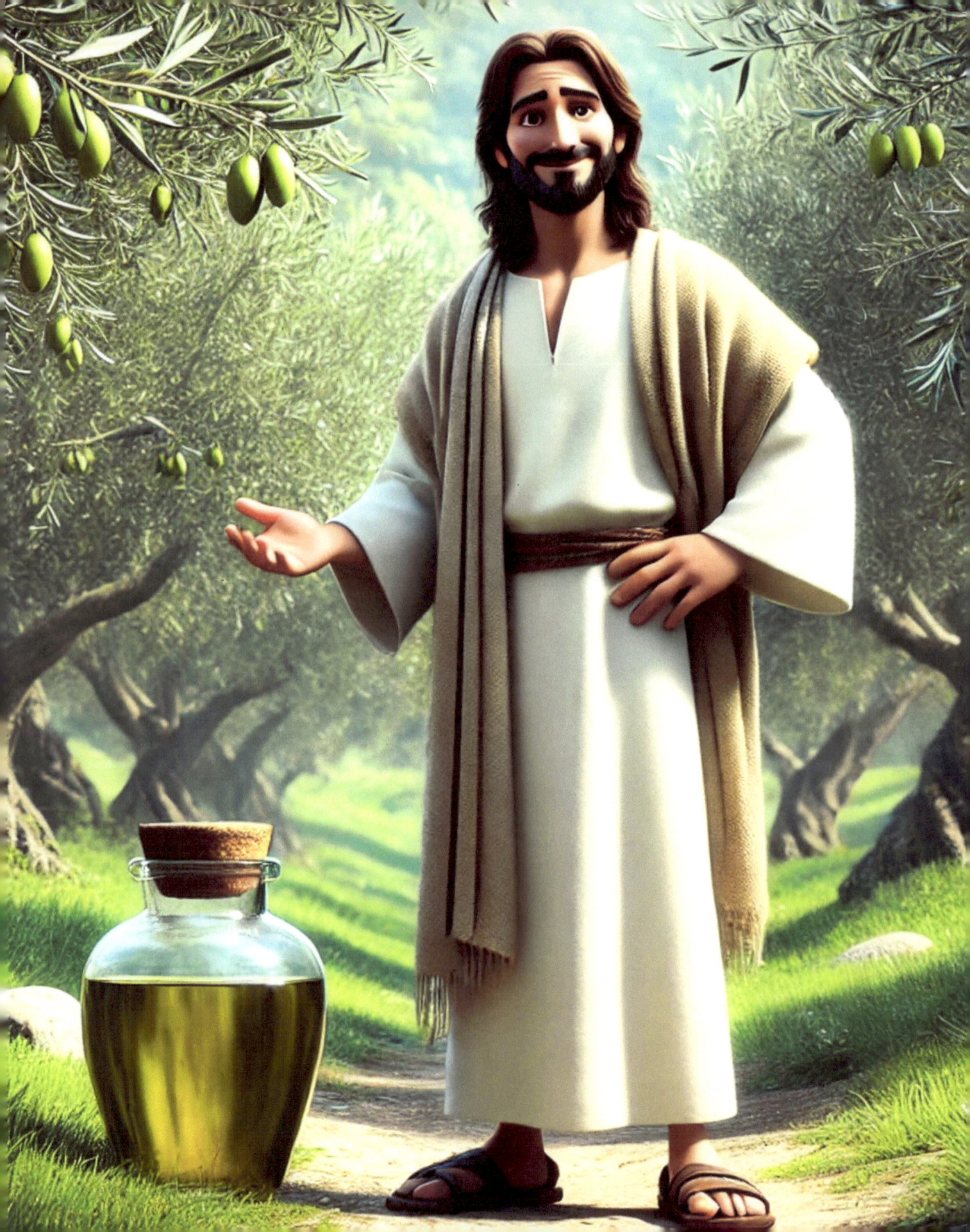

God made olive oil,
smooth and gold.

Healthy fats to keep
your body bold.

It helps your heart,
your brain, your skin—

A drizzle of goodness,
pure within!

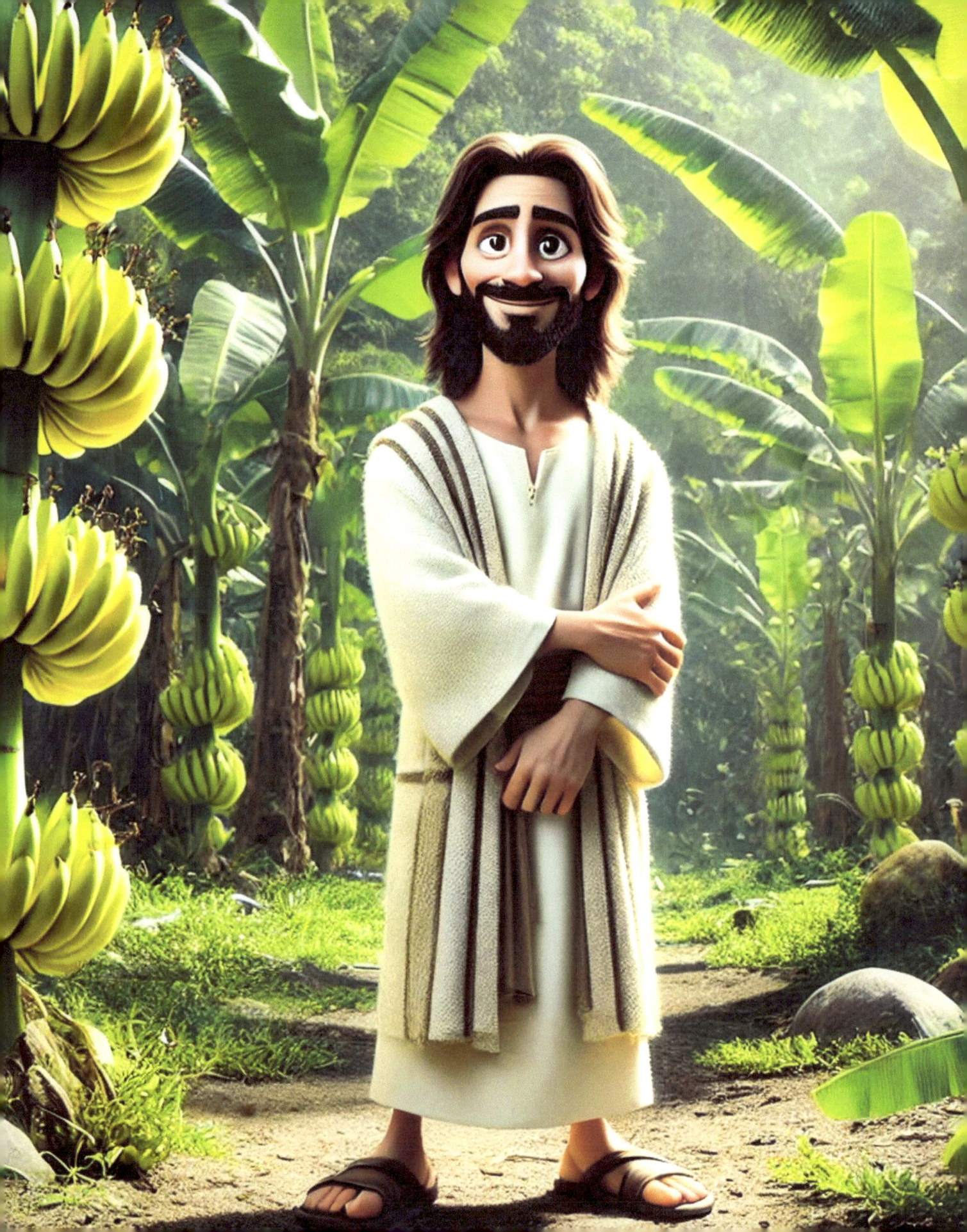

God made bananas,
yellow and sweet.

A potassium-packed
and easy treat.

They keep your
muscles working fine—

So you can climb
and feel divine!

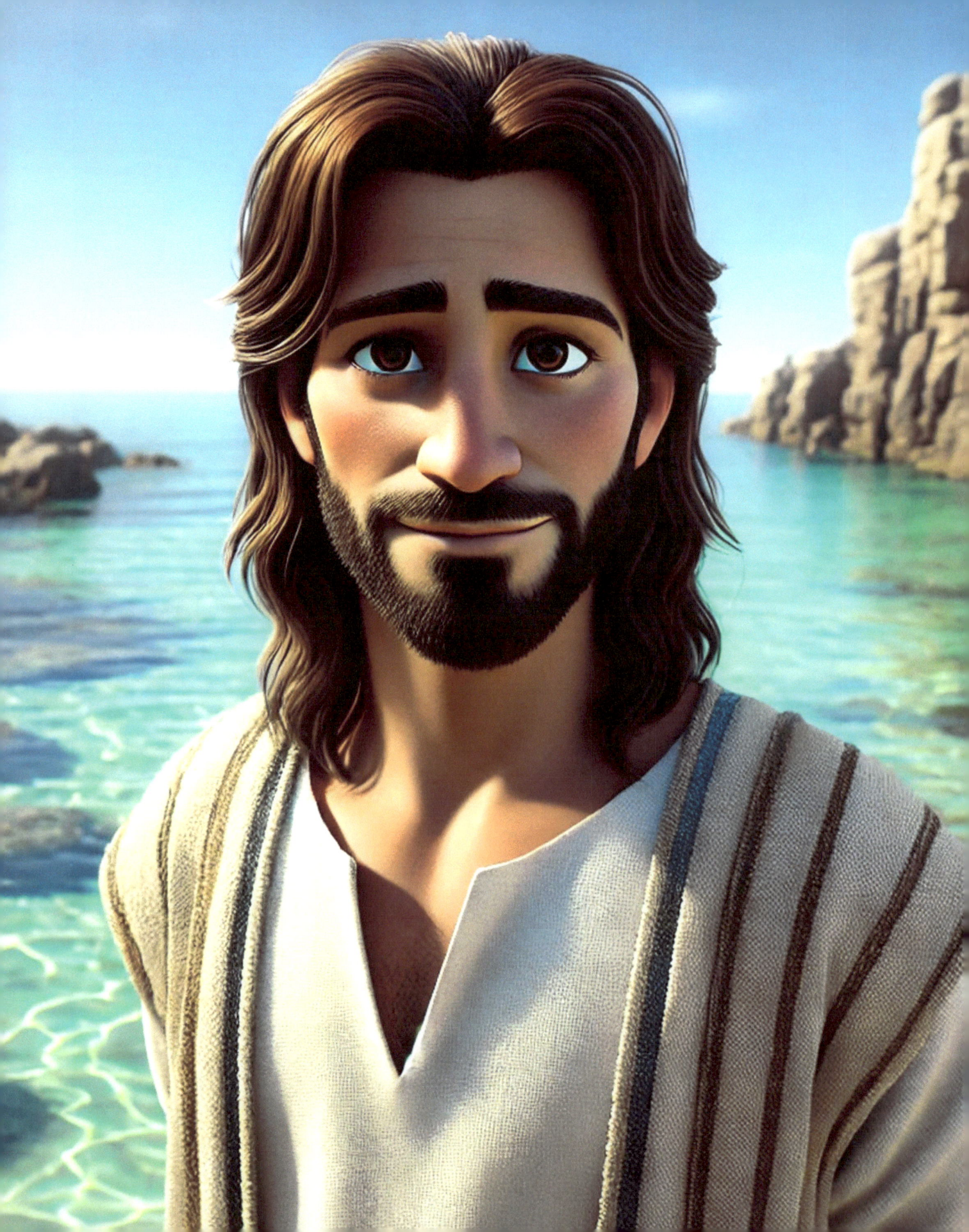

God made oceans,
vast and deep.

Full of treasures
that we reap.

Fish and seaweed,
food galore.

The oceans give us
health and more!

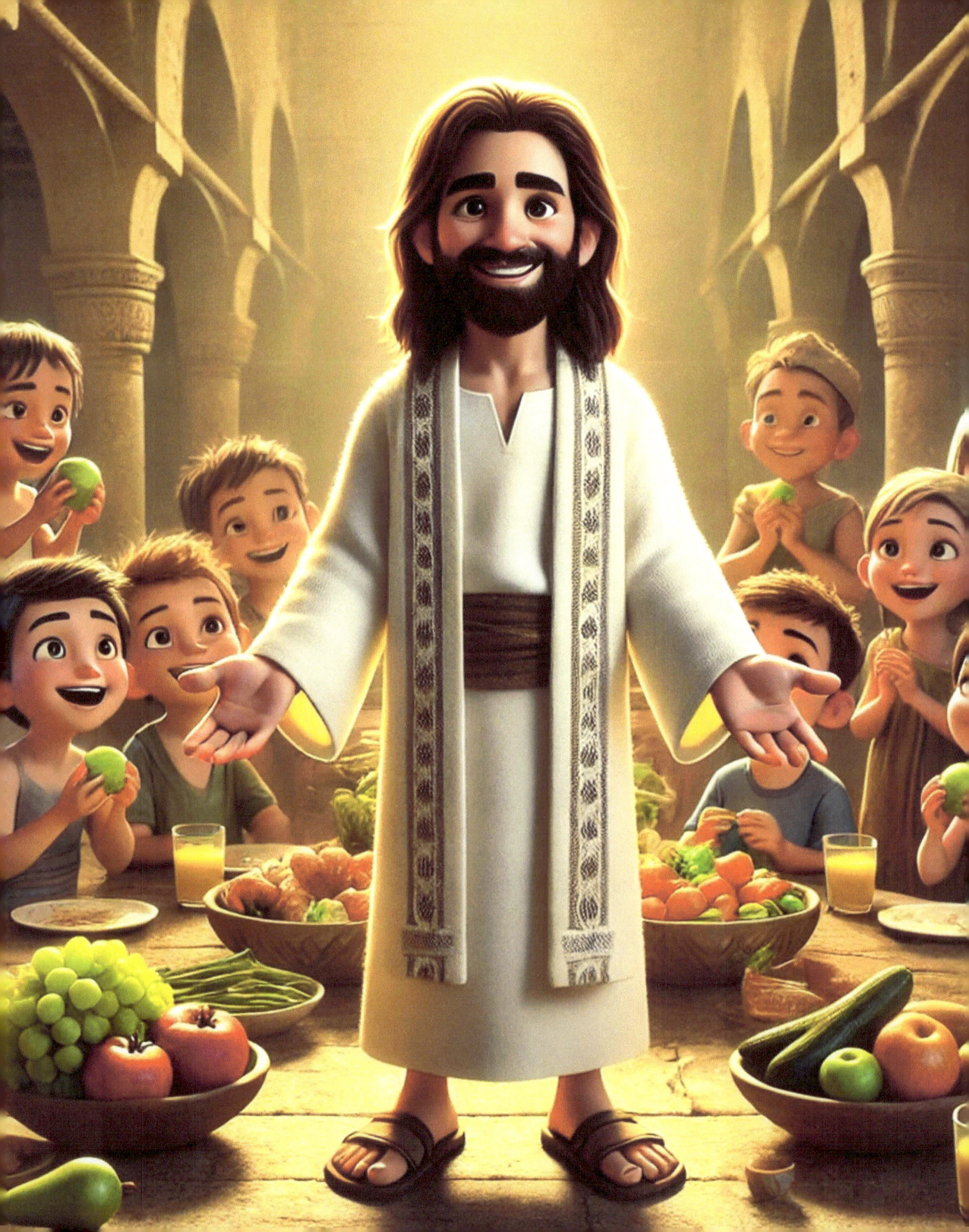

God made
everything we need.

To help us grow
in thought and deed.

Every bite is
a gift, you see.

A blessing for
you and me!

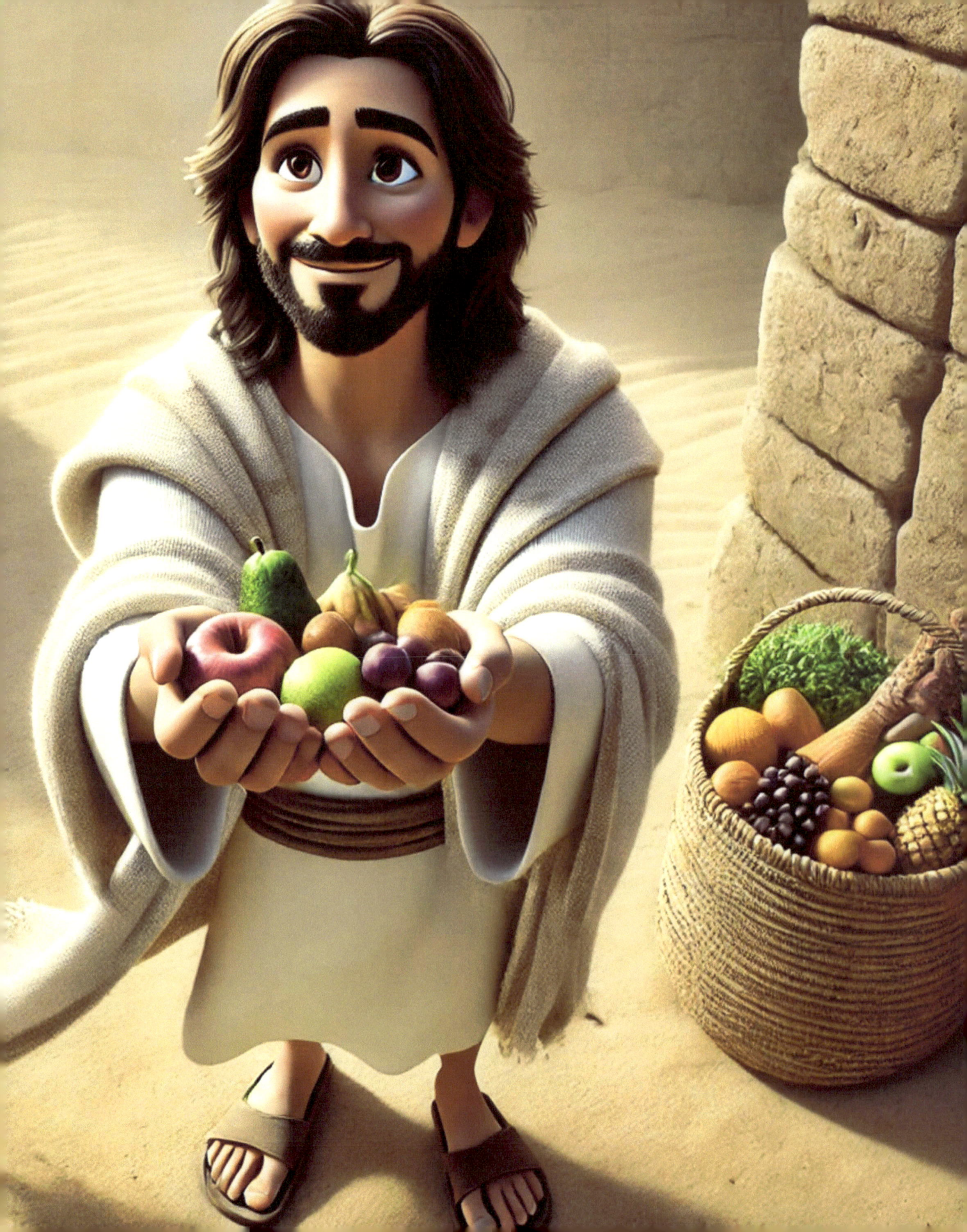

God made you,
so wonderfully bright.

A body to care for,
both day and night.

Fill it with good things,
share His love too.

The world is brighter
because of YOU!

Word Search

```
S P I N A C H D S C J M G D P A P K
S F N W O L I V E K P L H H K U E V
U Z D A T V U Z G D O E F O W D R R
N B M B H G S P V R R C P V N R K W
W A T E R E D L Z N A R H P F E X I
L N X N B O R E M X N V L I E I Y Z
J A G C R I C B C G G A O M C R S C
K N B E A N S C S W E P X C O K Y H
H A H H I W D L O V E P J I A E E A
Z L Y S O I L K O L N L Y K T D G N
T N C A R R O T B H I E M T J Y O G
I N U T S Z B L U E B E R R Y A K B
```

APPLE	CHICKEN	ORANGE
AVOCADO	EGG	PEPPER
BANANA	FISH	SOIL
BEANS	HERBS	SPINACH
BLUEBERRY	HONEY	SUN
BROCCOLI	NUTS	WATER
CARROT	OLIVE	

Fun Facts

- Did you know? Apples can float in water because they are made up of 25% air!

- An orange isn't always orange! Some oranges stay green, even when they're ripe.

- Bananas are berries too! And they grow in big groups called 'hands.'

- Carrots weren't always orange—they can also be purple, yellow, or even white!

- Bees visit over 1,000 flowers to make just one tiny drop of honey!

- Plants love dirt because it's full of food for their roots—like vitamins for them!

For more activites based on this book,

visit karattmultimedia.com

www.ingramcontent.com/pod-product-compliance
Lightning Source LLC
LaVergne TN
LVHW072129070426
835513LV00002B/40

9781971047003